# DR. DANIEL CASS-FUCHS

# Health Basics 101

*A Beginner's Guide To Staying Healthy*

# Contents

# Introduction

Welcome to Health Basics 101 - a beginner's guide to understanding and improving your health. Good health is essential for a happy and fulfilling life, but with so much information out there, it can be overwhelming and confusing to know where to start. That's where this guide comes in - we'll cover the basics of what you need to know to take control of your health and well-being.

In this guide, we'll discuss the importance of good nutrition, exercise, sleep, and mental health, as well as provide tips and tricks to help you make simple, positive changes in your lifestyle. We'll also cover the basics of managing chronic conditions, preventing illness, and navigating the healthcare system.

Whether you're a complete health newbie or just looking to refresh your knowledge, Health Basics 101 has something for everyone. So, let's get started on the path to a healthier you!

# Contraceptive Pills and It's Problems (Contraception )

Contraception is the control of ripeness to forestall pregnancy.

Prophylactic is any specialist that diminishes the probability of origination

### REASONS OF CONTRACEPTION

1. To forestall ovulation in a lady

2. To prevent sperm from meeting an ovum in the Fallopian tube to forestall preparation.

3. To keep a prepared ovum from embedding in the uterus (belly).

## Preventive Methods

These contraception strategies could be complete (long-lasting) or intermittent forbearance (evasion) from sex between the couple.

# Natural Method

This is the technique for staying away from pregnancy (origination) in light of endeavors to pinpoint a lady's rich period around the hour of ovulation; with the goal that sex can be kept away from as of now or controlled.

### *TYPES OF NATURAL METHODS ARE AS FOLLOWS:*

## *Calendar Method*

The scheduling strategy under ovulation depends on the monthly cycle of a lady by which counting is finished from the first day of the lady's feminine stream (time frame) till between the twelfth to the fourteenth day to determine her ovulation period since it is ovulation time that the lady can become pregnant. Subsequently, the couple should not engage in sexual relations from the ninth to the twelfth day, and between the thirteenth day to the fifteenth day, the chance of becoming pregnant is extremely high while the sixteenth day is to make recompense in case of any hormonal change or a day postpone in ovulation event, just no doubt. Then, at that point, every other day is free till the start of the following feminine progression of the lady (spouse).

## *Ovulation Temperature Thermometer Strategy*

Temperature is one more strategy to decide on ovulation. This strategy depends on the typical ascent of a lady's internal heat level. During ovulation, the temperature of a lady isn't steady. Consequently, an ovulation thermometer ought to be utilized after her ovulation to decide the stability of her temperature day to day. Sex is viewed as protected provided that there has been a supported temperature increase for something like 3 days. It is as of now, the couple is allowed to have intercourse when the temperature of the lady is at a steady or typical temperature rate.

## Cervical Mucus Method

Another strategy to decide ovulation is the cervical bodily fluid technique. This technique is otherwise called the charging strategy, by which the couple endeavors to pinpoint the ripe time of the lady by noticing and diagramming the sum and presence of cervical bodily fluid during the monthly cycle. You should have the option to perceive the progressions in the amount and the presence of the bodily fluid before ovulation and frequently at ovulation legitimate.

## The Symptothermal Method

This is the mix of ovulation thermometer temperature checks and the perception of the cervical bodily fluid strategy.

## Withdrawal Method Or Coitus Interruptus Method

This is the cycle, by which the spouse, immediately pulls out or hauls his penis out from the vaginal of the wife prior to delivering his sperm during sex. Only one out of every odd man can stand to adapt to this strategy since certain men might stand by till they show up at climax and right now when they at long last pull out their penis from the vaginal some limited quantity of sperm has probably been kept or dropped into the vaginal obscure to them. Few out of every odd man or spouse can adapt to this technique. This technique is for developing disapproval of men or spouses. It isn't for child spouses.

# Hormonal Method

In this strategy, the ladies utilize manufactured progesterone drugs, which are frequently joined with engineered estrogens to forestall pregnancy. These medications stifle ovulation, and it makes cervical bodily fluid thick and impervious to sperm. These medications likewise cause the diminishing of the covering of the belly to lessen the possibility of a prepared egg from embedding effectively. The chemicals can likewise be given as preventative inserts under the skins, by infusion, or be delivered by IUD-intrauterine gadgets.

# Obstruction or Barrier Method

This is the utilization of a gadget as well as a synthetic to prevent sperm from arriving at an ovum to forestall treatment and pregnancy.

Hindrance techniques likewise help the counteraction of physically communicated infections like AIDS, genital herpes, viral hepatitis, gonorrhea, and so on. For preventative hindrance strategies, the male condom is one of the most broadly utilized boundary contraceptives. Female condoms are like male condoms yet bigger than male condoms

Other female hindrance techniques incorporate the stomach - a hemispherical vault of flimsy elastic with a metal spring in the edge to hold it set up against the vaginal wall, impeding the entry to the cervix. It is utilized with a spermicide.

A cervical cap is an option in contrast to the stomach. The preventative wipe, which is a dispensable, round, polyurethane froth wipe impregnated with spermicide, is embedded profound into the vaginal and left set up for no less than 6 hours after sex (intercourse). Spermicides, as spray froths, creams, gels, and pessaries are set in the vaginal as close as conceivable to the cervix presently before sex (intercourse). A few spermicides ought not to be utilized with elastic boundary gadgets. (Directions are typically composed on the name, read it) mechanical and synthetic means utilized together accurately can be profoundly successful in forestalling pregnancy.

## Preventative Implant Method

This is a sort of hormonal strategy for contraception where long-acting preventative medications are embedded under the skin. An embed comprises a little pole that consistently delivers a progesterone drug into the circulatory system of the lady every once in a while.

## Preventative Inject-able Method

This is likewise a hormonal strategy for contraception in which long-acting progesterone drugs are given by infusion each 2 to 90 days.

Inject-able contraceptives are exceptionally compelling however may cause feminine aggravations, weight gain, cerebral pains, and sickness (regurgitating) or having the sentiments to upchuck, particularly during the initial not many long stretches of purpose. In the wake of halting the utilization of preventative infusions or oral prophylactic medications, it requires between a half year to 1 year for a lady that has been on preventative to become pregnant. The delay is for the framework of the lady to regularize itself. Better actually see a clinical specialist for assessment before it is past the point of no return.

# Preventative Emergency Method

This is an action, taken to keep away from pregnancy following unprotected sex. For this situation, there are two primary techniques. The hormonal and actual techniques. For the hormonal strategy, the morning after sex, an oral preventative pill ought to be accepted in a high portion quickly after unprotected sex, ideal in no less than 12 hours, but not later than (72 hours) 3 days subsequently. The pills contain a high portion of progesterone. (E.g I-pill preventative tablet).

In the actual strategy for crisis prophylactic technique, an IUD (intrauterine gadget) is embedded by a clinical specialist in no less than 5 days of unprotected sex. The two strategies are remembered to work by keeping a prepared egg from embedding in the belly (uterus).

# Coil Method

The curl technique is otherwise called IUD or IUCD, meaning - intrauterine prophylactic gadget.

The curl technique is a mechanical gadget that is embedded into the belly or uterus as contraception to forestall pregnancy. Most IUDs are plastic gadgets with one or the other copper or silver consolidated to work on their viability. One sort of IUD delivers limited quantities of progesterone hormones and is here and there known as an intrauterine system (IUS). The curl strategy forestalls the implantation of a prepared egg in the mass of the belly or uterus. The curl is embedded through the vaginal and cervix into the belly hole or space. Once ready, an IUD gives quick security. Most IUDs have a plastic string joined to make expulsion more straightforward and to show its presence when set up. IUDs should be supplanted following 3 to 10 years, contingent upon the sort. Ladies who have been pregnant are more averse to inconveniences than ladies who have never been pregnant. For instance, they might encounter less torment on inclusion and have a lighter feminine stream and lower ejection rates. IUDs are generally not suggested for ladies with fibroid or an unpredictable uterine (belly) hole. In the event that the feminine stream is weighty or there is a set of experiences or expanded chance of Pelvic Inflammatory Disease (PID), a progesterone IUD might be suggested.

IUDs only here and there cause issues and can be taken out.

Non-Progestin IUDs or curl expands the gamble of pelvic fiery infection (PID), which can prompt extremely durable fruitlessness. An uncommon entanglement of IUD use is the hole of the uterus (openings in the belly), which most regularly happens at the hour of inclusion of the loop or IUD. Intrauterine framework (IUS) is a mechanical preventative gadget that looks like an IUD yet in addition contains the progesterone hormone levonorgestrel.

The IUS gadget is fitted inside the uterus (belly), where the chemical is delivered gradually and ceaselessly for as long as 5 years. The IUS additionally forestalls pregnancy by influencing the uterine coating and thickening the cervical bodily fluid.

Notwithstanding its prophylactic impacts. It makes feminine periods lighter. It could be utilized for ladies with weighty periods or weighty streams (menorrhagia)

## Oral Contraceptive Method

A gathering of oral medications arrangements containing at least one engineered female sex hormone, taken by ladies in a month-to-month cycle to forestall pregnancy.

### *TYPES OF ORAL CONTRACEPTIVES*

There are two significant classes of oral prophylactic pills.

## Consolidated Pill Or Phased Pill

This oral preventative pill is generally alluded to as joined pill or staged pill since it contained both estrogen drugs and progestogen drug fixings.

Estrogen pills contain ethinylestradiol while progestogen pills contain levonorgestrel and norethisterone.

When utilized accurately, the quantity of pregnancies among ladies involving oral contraceptives for one year is under 1%. Genuine disappointment rates might be multiple times higher, especially for the small pill, which must be taken at definitively a similar time every day.

Consolidated pills or staged pills build estrogen and progesterone levels. This hormonal level increment meddles or forestalls the development of two hormones called, luteinizing hormone (LH) and follicle-stimulating hormone (FSH), which thus forestalls ovulation. Estrogen-containing pills offer insurance against uterine or belly malignant growth, ovarian disease, ovarian sores, endometriosis, and iron inadequacy pallor.

They additionally will more often than not make feminine periods lighter, standard, and generally torment-free.

### SIDE EFFECTS OF CONSOLIDATED CONTRACEPTIVE PILLS

Conceivable incidental effects incorporate sickness (spewing), weight gain, wretchedness, enlarged bosoms, diminished sex drive, increment hunger, leg cramps, stomach issues, cerebral pains, and tipsiness. These pills may likewise irritate coronary illness or cause hypertension, gallstones, jaundice, and seldom, liver disease, the hazard of bosom malignant growth. All the more genuinely, there is a gamble of apoplexy (blood clump in the vein, consequently making bloodstream unthinkable) causing a stroke or a pneumonic embolism (obstructing of a conduit that supplies blood to the lungs e.g blood cluster, fat globules, air bubble). Consolidated or staged pills might slow down milk creation and ought not to be taken during bosom taking care of taking care of.

## Mini Pill

A mini pill is a sort of oral prophylactic which contains just a progestogen drug. The scaled-down pill works predominantly by making the bodily fluid covering the cervix excessively thick to be infiltrated by sperm. Certain medications can disable or forestall the viability of oral prevention.

### SIDE EFFECTS OF MINI PILL

All oral contraceptives can cause draining between periods, particularly the mini pill. Other conceivable unfriendly impacts of the mini pill incorporate sporadic feminine periods, ectopic pregnancy, ovarian sores, and so forth.

**If it's not too much trouble, TAKE NOTE OF THIS**

Estrogen-based pills like the joined pills ought to for the most part be kept away from ladies with hypertension, elevated cholesterol or having a lot of fat in the circulation system, liver illness, headache, otosclerosis (hearing issue or deafness), or who are at expanded hazard of apoplexy (blood cluster). They are not typically endorsed to ladies with individual or family backgrounds of heart or circulatory problems, or who experience unexplained vaginal dying. The small-scale pill or a low estrogen pill might be utilized by ladies who ought to stay away from estrogens. Bosom taking care of moms ought to mind the sort of preventative pill they drink since they needn't bother with the joined pill.

# Flat Belly ( How To Avoid Big Tummy)

Nowadays numerous teens, young women, ladies, and men are growing large stomachs on a regular schedule, because of their propensities or way of life.

The accompanying circumstances underneath, if stringently followed, will assist with managing the issue of a major paunch.

To keep a level stomach or need to lessen your generally huge midsection these circumstances will enormously assist you with accomplishing that reason.

1. Keep away from food varieties that you might be adversely affected by or that you know as a matter of fact disturbs you. In the event that you have a frail stomach-related framework and feel swollen and weighty after dinner, you can take stomach-related chemical tablets with the feast.

Continuously bite your food gradually and completely as processing starts with spit blended in with food in the mouth, with the assistance of the salivary synthetic called ptyalin.  As individuals progress in years, the creation of hydrochloric corrosives from the stomach frequently becomes deficient for the proficient absorption of proteins. This can be overwhelmed by tasting a little glass of water containing one to two teaspoons of apple juice vinegar drink with each feast.

The most well-known food varieties to cause gastrointestinal peevish gut conditions are gluten or dairy items for example milk, margarine, cheddar, cream, and frozen yogurt.

This is on the grounds that these food varieties contain receptive proteins and lactose. Many individuals feel substantially less swelled when they keep away from these food sources. Try not to ingest too much espresso.

2. Try not to eat on the off chance that you feel worried or restless. Doing this might influence your bloodstream and redirect it from the digestive tracts and liver to different regions of the body. Eating right now will prompt stomach bulging and unfortunate assimilation.

3. Pay attention to your body. Try not to eat when you are not hungry. Have a piece of natural product, a little part of a vegetable plate of mixed greens, or a glass of water all things considered.

Try not to put your dinners nonstop - that is, while eating turns into a planned propensity and individuals will eat say by 8:00 am, 1:00 pm and 7:00 pm separately, come downpour or daylight, hunger or not.

It is a lot better to put your feast times around your craving similarly kids do and pay less notice to the clock. In the event that you are prone to eating ordinary feasts when you are not eager your liver will be working excessively hard and will endure with restrictive mileage, very much like abused joint inflammation joints.

4. Try not to eat a lot of sugar, particularly refined sugars, as this will be changed over into an undesirable sort of fat called fatty oil. Many individuals become fat on a low-fat, high-carbs diet and this causes the stomach to get greater.

5. Keep away from fake sugars, aspartame is tracked down in diet colas, a few sodas pops, and a few diabetic food varieties and can cause hypoglycemia (low sugar level in the body) and weakness (sleepiness). In the event that you

want something sweet, utilize new crude organic products, sun-dried natural products, or stevia (a normally sweet spice).

6. Stay away from clogging by eating a lot of crude organic products, what's more, vegetables and drinking a little measure of water it spans. Tasting water at stretches assists with purging the liver and kidney and helps weight reduction. Drinking an excess of water while eating can lessen these nutrients and supplements.

Keep away from a lot of liquid or water with dinners (while eating, drink less).

Crude products of the soil contain nutrients, minerals, and phytonutrients that are great for cell restoration and collagen development in the body.

7. Keep away from cholesterol or soaked fat, since it is fit for hurting the liver in the event that it is being consumed routinely. For example, spread, huge cheddar, and so forth.

This immersed fat is equipped for influencing the size of the paunch adversely.

8. Try not to eat late hours of the evening and weighty food varieties. Your lunch can be weighty food with the goal that it can last a very long time before night.

9. Stay away from sodas, and frozen yogurt, stay away from drinks with much gas, sweet food sources, and handle natural product juice. All things considered, go for normal natural products that don't include synthetic compounds. The majority of these organic juice products in the market are simple mixes of sugar, water, flavor, variety, trans fat (added substance), other synthetic fixings, and so on. Assuming that you want natural product juice drinks, you ought to go for those that are produced using regular natural products or set them up without help from anyone else. Zobo drink is great

for you since it contains ginger and now and again garlic and other normal fixings.

10. Try not to eat a lot of red meat (hamburger) all things being equal, eat fish. Even better, you can go for white meat like chicken or turkey, and so on, however not to eat in abundance. Bear in mind that the majority of these frozen food varieties are not great for your well-being in view of the additive synthetic compounds utilized.

11. Decrease the abundance corrosive in your midsection to try not to make it greater

12. The utilization of support. This includes the tying of a covering, material, or wide belt around the stomach or midsection for longer hours every once in a while as different circumstances are being noticed.

13. Stay away from cocktails like a lager, hot beverages, and so on. All things considered, go for non-alcoholic wine.

14. Eat earthy colored rice for example mom gold rice, imperial steed rice, and so on. They are great for you yet keep away from white rice, noodles, and so on. Quite a bit of it will cause you a major paunch.

15. At spans accept vitamin B-perplexing as a food supplement in light of its capabilities to the body. Vitamin B-1 (known as thiamine) helps for the versatility of the nerves, muscles, tendons, muscles, and so on. Stay away from white sugar whether in blocks or powder structure since it bothers the enormous midsection. All things considered, go for regular honey or earthy-colored sugar and no sugars.

16. Keep away from low-quality foods like meat pie, cake, jawline jaw, donuts, rolls, hot dog rolls, and so forth.

17 Deworm yourself at regular intervals. Purchase combatrin (pyrantel pamoate) medication to drink like clockwork to annihilate the excess worms of all classes in your stomach. Worms are parasites and they are damaging to our tummies and the whole body framework.

# Fibroid Growth

A fibroid is quite possibly the deadliest illness that influences ladies. Research shows that 40% of ladies have fibroid or an extremely high inclination to it. It unleashes destruction on the belly of the person in question or victim and when it develops, it leaves torments.

A fibroid is a sluggish developing, noncancerous harmless cancer of the belly (uterus), comprising smooth muscle and connective tissue.

There might be at least 1 fibroid development, and they might be pretty much as little as a pea or as extensive as a grapefruit.

There are various sorts of fibroid. Fibroid development can spread all around the belly over the long haul on the off chance that care isn't taken. Fibroid development could be solitary or numerous fibroid. This relies upon the term (season) of the development. The manner in which plantain or banana trees or sucker sprouts (develop) and spread over a space of land is the same way fibroid spreads.

Any fibroid casualty shouldn't underestimate it or kid about it. It is better in the event that it is taken out on time. It is smarter to eliminate it than to consider ingesting a few medications to contract it. Contracting implies that the fibroid is still there, however developing at a sluggish rate. This could be perilous while perhaps not appropriately observed. The most ideal choice is complete expulsion of the fibroid development.

Keep to your clinic arrangement until it is at last taken out. Fibroid are normal, showing up most frequently in ladies between the ages of 25 to 45 years. The reason is believed to be connected with an unusual reaction of the estrogen hormones. Oral contraceptives containing estrogen can make fibroid expand as can pregnancy. Diminished estrogen creation after menopause ordinarily makes fibroid development shrivel.

On the off chance that a fibroid is developed, it projects into the hole of the belly (uterus), it might cause a weighty feminine stream or delayed feminine periods e.g having a feminine stream past 8 days to up to 10 or 14 days which is unusual.

A huge fibroid might apply strain on the bladder, causing regular passing of pee, or on the entrails, causing spinal pain or clogging.

Fibroid that twist the uterine pit (belly) might be liable for repetitive unnatural birth cycles or fruitlessness in ladies. Fibroid that don't cause side effects are in many cases found during a routine pelvic assessment. Ultrasound examination can affirm the finding of fibroid development. The clinical medical procedure is expected for fibroid that cause serious side effects.

At times they can be eliminated with hysteroscopy or under broad sedation, leaving the belly in salvageable shape.

In a circumstance where the fibroid patient didn't deal with the fibroid development on time, in the event that it is found restorative that the fibroid development has impacted or obliterated the belly, the main answer to save the existence of the fibroid patient is to eliminate the belly alongside the fibroid development.

That sort of activity is called "hysterectomy".

# Signs And Symptoms Of Fibroid

1. Sporadic monthly cycle

2. Delayed feminine stream

3. Weighty feminine stream (now and again with cluster)

4. Expanded recurrence of pee (micturition)

5. Criticality of pee

6. Midsection torment going from gentle to serious

7. Spinal pain

8. Blockage

9. There may likewise be stomach distension (extended midsection).

10. There might be a general sensation of substantialness

11. Pelvic uneasiness or torment.

# Complications of Fibroid

On the off chance that fibroid development isn't dealt with or gone to on time, it can cause or prompt the accompanying issues:

1. Unsuccessful labor of Pregnancy. As the fibroid development possesses the depression of the belly, there will be not adequate room and, surprisingly, enough blood and supplements for the hatchling (child) to get by. It is in

uncommon cases that a few ladies become pregnant and can bring forth the youngsters alive on the grounds that the fibroid has not completely developed to estimate or, more than likely there will be complexities or unnatural birth cycle.

Any lady that has fibroid development ought to take care of business prior to considering pregnancy to keep away from unforeseen conditions.

2. Extreme frailty. The deficiency of dark red (platelets), as the fibroid, benefits from the blood of the lady.

3. Fibroid causes fruitlessness, which might be essential or auxiliary fruitlessness.

4. Fibroid development can cause passing while possibly not appropriately made due.

## Instructions to Avoid Fibroid

The accompanying practices can bother fibroid development.

Accordingly, females ought to attempt however much as could be expected to stay away from such.

1. Reliance on oral prophylactic pills (particularly those that contained estrogen). An illustration of such a pill is the consolidated or staged pill.

2. Aseptic early termination (unhygienic, frequently criminal early termination).

3. The over consumption of greasy food varieties that are high in cholesterol.

4. Postponed cyesis (pregnancy). At the point when a lady has postponed pregnancy for quite a while, for the most part traversing years. To that end, fibroid development is normal among ladies who are above mid-twenties upwards between 25 to 45 years old. The chemicals that would have sustained the advancement of the embryo (unborn youngster) may advance fibroid assuming pregnancy is missing over an extensive stretch. Presently, there have not been many instances of females before 25 years old experiencing fibroid development. This calls for alertness in our propensities and ways of life.

5. Late marriage rehearses advanced fibroid. This is one reason a few societies advocate early marriage (say 18 years or more), and childbearing by women of childbearing age for their spouses.

6. Inordinate liquor admission which might up the muscle versus fat level because of unhealthy substances.

7. Cigarette smoking solidifies the veins, subsequently restraining blood flow

8. Ineffectively oversaw disease in the female regenerative framework.

# Types Of Fibroid

## Intramural Fibroid

This kind of fibroid development is situated inside the belly (uterus). It could be available in the belly without clear side effects until it is extremely enormous prior to displaying side effects.

## Subserosal Fibroid

This sort of fibroid becomes underneath the peritoneal surface of the belly (uterus). It can get exceptionally huge. Most times, a subserosal fibroid might turn out to be highly parasitic, reliably prospering through the chemicals delivered typically by the body of the lady. To that end, fibroid will generally shrivel when a lady clocks menopause time of between 45 to 55 years due to an absence of a satisfactory estrogen chemical stockpile at that stage

## Submucosal Fibroid

This sort of fibroid is situated in the muscle underneath the endometrium (the mucous layer lining) of the belly. Submucosal fibroid twists (ruins) the state of the belly.

The development might prompt extreme dying, particularly during the times of the feminine stream and this is normally answerable for confusion, for example, serious weakness because of weighty dying, barrenness, and passing, while perhaps not appropriately made due.

## Cervical Fibroid

This is a kind of fibroid development that is situated in the cervix (that is, the neck of the belly). It seldom happens and can likewise reach out to connecting structures.

# Treatment Of Fibroid

Clinical treatment of fibroid incorporates the organization of gonadorelin analogs. Little fibroid can be obliterated by diathermy utilizing a hysteroscope. Bigger ones might be coagulated by laparoscopic through a course of laparoscopic myolysis or eliminated by myomectomy or uterine corridor embolization, uterine supply route ligation. Any other way, a hysterectomy might be vital (expulsion of the belly).

On the off chance that uneasiness and different side effects are missing, a medical procedure isn't needed.

# Weak Penis Erection And The Solution

## Erection

This is the hardness, enlarging, and rise of the penis that happens because of sexual excitement or actual feeling. The erectile tissue of the penis loads up with blood as the veins in it enlarge. Muscles around vessels contract, what's more, prevent blood from passing on to the penis to keep an erection. A determined erection without even a trace of sexual craving is called priapism.

## Erectile Dysfunction Or Weak Erection

This is the failure of a man to accomplish or keep up with his penis erection to empower vaginal entrance for sex.

The circumstances where the course of penis erection is disturbed from accomplishing erection could be an incomplete disappointment or complete disappointment condition.

# Causes For Weak Erection

There are many causes and contributing variables, frequently a mix of actual causes and mental elements are liable for the condition.

## *Actual Causes*

1. Peripheral Vascular Disease

This is the restricting of veins in the body subsequently confining the typical bloodstream.  Fringe vascular illness is brought about by atherosclerosis - which is the solidifying of the veins by cholesterol (fats in the circulation system) additionally smoking.

2. Hypogonadism

This is the under activity of testicles or ovaries. Hypogonadism might be brought about by issues of the gonads(the sex organs - the testicles in men and the ovaries in ladies) or a problem of the pituitary gland that causes lacking creation of gonadotrophin hormones. Hypogonadism is just the lack of sex hormone discharge in the sex organ. In men hypogonadism causes androgen hormone inadequacy, making man's erection and sexual craving to be feeble and exhausting.

While it likewise causes the lack of estrogen in ladies in this way making the ladies not have affection for sex each time they are required for sex by their spouses.

3. Endocrine System problem

This system is the assortment of glands around the body that produces hormones like the thyroid, pancreas, testicles, ovaries, and adrenal glands. Any increment or decline in the creation of a particular hormone slows down the cycle it controls.

4. Physical irregularities or inward underlying deformities of the penis.

5. Certain drugs like hypertensive medications, drugs for stroke treatment, drugs for diabetes, and so on. Such medications diminish sexual inclinations and thus influence penis erection.

6. Diabetes Mellitus' abundance of sugar in the circulatory system influences adversely how much blood is accessible for dissemination or stream to the testicles. It causes fatigue and shortcomings.

## Mental Causes

The mental variables influencing penile erection have to would with your conditions of care, like sexual memory, sentiments, considerations, and your overall discernment as well as your outside or actual conduct appearances.

For example, in the event that a man isn't in the right temper (in a positive state of mind), his penis erection will be feeble or contorted.

## Treatment And Prevention

### Drugs

Certain medications help to increment blood flow to the cavernous sinuses (somewhere within) the penis to cause an erection. Such medications are normally gulped 1 hour before sex while one of the most commonest brand names or (market name) is Viagra. (We have USA Viagra and Nigeria kinds of Viagra. The USA kind of Viagra is all the more remarkable and powerful. The synthetic name of Viagra is called sildenafil). There is additionally the inject-able one called alprostadil.

Its aftereffects for certain individuals are dazedness, slight migraine, and sickness.

## Take Multivitamins And Mineral Supplements

Numerous men don't drink or take mineral enhancements and blood medication like Omega H3, Astymin, B-complex, Calcium, Astyfer, Bunto, Vitamin C, Ranferon-12, and so forth.

These items and numerous others help to renew the body and fix broken-down tissues of the body framework. Most men are lacking in these minerals, nutrients, and amino acids. Such lacks influence the elements of the body system adversely. These enhancements help to decide the strength or endurance of a man and in this way reflect how far he can go physically in addition to other things.

It requires 21 days medicinally for any man to recapture, recharge or supplant the sperm he has delivered during each sex.

3. Evasion of many sodas and sweet things by and large. Those bundled juice in packs, jars, and jugs practically 100 percent of them contain a lot of gas, sugar, and synthetic added substances which help to delay or broaden the time frame of realistic usability of those items on the lookout, with the goal that the items won't lapse on time.

These synthetic added substances and sugar influence the body's capabilities.

4. Satisfactory rest and enough rest are great variables for each man's sexual great exhibition.

Sluggishness and absence of satisfactory rest are serious issues relieving penis erection because of STRESS.

Men ought to figure out how to rest their body frameworks and rest for an adequate number of hours 6 to 8 hours endorsed medicinally to revive or renew their lost energy or strength before going into sex with their spouses. Stress disappoints the sexual presentation and fulfillment of any man independent old enough.

Stress kills sex drive and want. Attempt however much as could reasonably be expected to keep away from pressure. 70% of hitched ladies despise their marriage or spouses physically due to erection brokenness. Restoratively, it takes a lady between 15 to 20 minutes to climax under typical circumstances when the spouse knows the ideal locations to contact or sentiment her. A few men can be with their spouses for 2 hours or more without having the option to invigorate or excite them. Then spouses ought to have the option to request their wives what and which region from their bodies invigorates them quickly so they can do equity to it and support or satisfy their wives. Along these lines, spouses ought to figure out which region of the husband's body invigorates them better to keep the husband on top till endlessness. Those that are now doing great ought to enhance it with understanding.

5. Men need to eat right and as at when due. Eat great food that you will get supplements from. Likewise, hydrate day to day somewhere around 8 ordinary glass cups of water to improve your body's liquid. Lessen overabundance of liquor consumption. Eat normal natural products like nursery egg, pecans, cashew nut, orange, pawpaw, carrot, pineapple, banana, cucumber, plantain, watermelon, and vegetables routinely.

Eat a lot of fish no less than two times every week and decrease how much meat you do eat.

Two times every week get a few new severe passes on to get them into a cup, add some salt to it, and drink it. It is awesome and therapeutic for your whole body's capabilities.

6. Keep away from regular jungle fever assaults.

A man that is generally tired of intestinal sickness (fever) can not perform physically. He will continuously be having the issue of a powerless erection prompting dis-satisfactory sex. The explanation is that the blood flow to the penis and gonads won't be sufficiently adequate to control the penis erection as the intestinal sickness disease benefits from the red platelets of the person in question. This prompts the debilitating of the body frameworks and the mental capabilities which thus influences the erection of a man adversely.

7. Sexually transmitted infection can likewise cause a powerless erection of the penis.

An intermittent or extensive stretch of untreated physically communicated diseases harms the testicles and causes blockage of the penis tubes and so forth.

Hence, don't sit around idly treating any disease that is analyzed for you in the emergency clinic.

8. To keep a decent penis erection, the spouse should assume her part (rather than resting like a log of wood on the bed) she ought to be contacting (romancing) her significant other delicately as the man infiltrates to keep the erection of the penis dynamic.

In any case, in the event that the spouse doesn't have her impact in such a manner the man's erection will begin running down and discharge will take action accordingly.

In this way, during the demonstration of sex the spouse should not yield or be bashful, she ought to be contacting the areola of the husband, head, back, ears, and bottom, and kiss him to keep the penis erect and working in the vaginal. Many spouses whose spouses don't contact or sentiment them during the demonstration of sex generally have frail erections during the demonstration of sex. This is incomplete in the event that the spouse doesn't respond to the sentiment with the wife moreover.

# Quick Ejaculations And The Solutions

Ejaculation is the emanation or the arrival of semen (sperm) from the penis at the climax. In no time before discharge, the muscles around the epididymides (the channels where sperm are put away), the prostate organ, and the fundamental vesicles contract musically, compelling the sperm from the epididymides to move advance and blend in with emissions from the original vesicles and prostate. At discharge, this liquid is expelled through the urethra and out of the body. Since both semen, what's more, pee leaves the body in a similar course, the bladder neck closes during discharge.

This doesn't just keep discharge from going into the bladder yet additionally prevents or keeps pee from polluting the semen. After every discharge, the bladder neck opens to permit pee entry or pec.

Fast discharge is a discharge irregularity or confusion which is a condition where the typical interaction or timing of discharge is upset inside the space of seconds or a few moments.

In untimely discharge, an emanation of semen happens previously or very quickly, following the entrance of the penis into the vaginal.

Untimely discharge is the most well-known sexual issue in men and is frequently because of over feeling or tension about sexual execution. In the event that the issue happens now and again, sexual guidance and strategies for deferring discharge might help.

# Prevention Of Quick Ejaculation

1.  As you infiltrate into the vaginal don't hurry to show that you are a superman or attempt to flaunt your muscles.  Be that as it may, abilities, well-being, and essentialness is required.

In this way, push in your penis tenderly and pull out prior to pushing in progressively once more.  Assuming that you proceed with this example now and then for some time your concern about speedy discharge will be addressed.

2. At the point when you saw that you are getting excessively animated during sex, you ought to rapidly decrease the rate at which you and your accomplice are stroking or romancing each other prior to proceeding again in pari-pasu.

3. During for-play before the demonstration of sex don't stand by till you are overcharged or over-animated prior to entering the vaginal. When your penis raises somewhat only approval for vaginal entrance. As the demonstration of sex is being finished, the penis will begin getting more flowed with blood.

4. During sex or as you infiltrate the vaginal your brain science is involved, simply free your psyche and focus on your sex accomplice since, in such a case that you don't think you might fantasize or let your memory (mind) redirect to another lady or woman you have been respecting elsewhere. In the event that you do, rather than your sex accomplice, the image of the weird woman will strike a chord as an impetus to overshoot your excitement to climax.

Thus, the result will be an untimely discharge. Likewise, assuming the spouse fantasized she will likewise encounter the resultant impact of speedy delivery (wet).

5. Try not to go into sex when hungry, on the grounds that it will make you frail and this can influence your discharge power and your penis erection

strength.

6. Take multivitamins and mineral enhancement occasionally to improve your body's capabilities and essentialness.

7. Stay away from much white sugar or sweet things like sodas, juice, frozen yogurt, and so on. Even better, you can go for earthy-colored sugar or normal honey for your food.

8. Keep away from disease. Men who experience the ill effects of an extensive stretch of untreated physically communicated diseases will generally experience the issue of untimely discharge more seriously than others.

9. Sluggishness is an absence of rest. At the point when you are worn out without sufficient rest prior to going into sex, it won't require your investment to rashly discharge.

This is the justification for why early morning sex is the best since you probably refreshed your nerves that control these feelings and discharge. Be that as it may, different circumstances as composed above ought to likewise be thought of as connecting early morning sex.

# Inhibited Ejaculation

This is a condition wherein penis erection is typical or even drawn out however discharge is truly challenging or unusually deferred or neglects to happen by any stretch of the imagination. The issue might be mental in the beginning, in which case directing may help, or it could be an entanglement of a problem like diabetes mellitus or liquor reliance. At times, repressed discharge happens as a result of specific medications like a few enemies of hypertensive and energizer drugs.

In retrograde discharge the valve at the base (neck) of the bladder which typically closes during discharge stays open and subsequently discharge is driven once again into the bladder. The retrograde discharge might happen because of a neurological illness, after a medical procedure on the bladder or prostatectomy (careful expulsion of the prostate organ).

There is no treatment, however, intercourse with a full bladder can in some cases bring about typical discharge.

# Ectopic And Molar Pregnancies(Pregnancy Abnormality)

## Ectopic Pregnancy

Is a pregnancy that occurs outside the belly (uterus), most normally in the Fallopian tube, but once in a while in the ovary or the stomach pit or cervix.

As the pregnancy creates, it might harm encompassing tissues, causing serious draining which is possibly hazardous and this requires crisis clinical treatment.

An ectopic pregnancy is brought about by the egg "losing" itself. In some cases, conditions like pelvic provocative sickness, Chlamydia, or gonorrhea can forestall the eggs' capacity to go through the Fallopian cylinder and settle or embed in the fitting spot. On the off chance that the treated egg isn't equipped for creating through the Fallopian tube because of the surprising state of the uterus (belly), Fallopian cylinder, or ovaries an ectopic pregnancy can happen.

## Causes for Ectopic Pregnancy

Ectopic pregnancy is more normal in ladies who have had past:

1. Pelvic inflammatory disease (PID)

2. The people who fix a few kinds of curl or intrauterine device (IUD) prophylactic boundary in their belly to forestall pregnancy.

3. The individuals who drink just progestogen oral preventative pills. Most ectopic pregnancies are found in the initial 2 months, frequently before the lady acknowledges she is pregnant.

## Symptoms Of Ectopic Pregnancy

Symptoms of ectopic pregnancy incorporate the following :

1. Severe pain in the lower mid-region

2. Vaginal bleeding

Inward bleeding may cause side effects of shock, whiteness (unusual pallor of the skin because of diminished blood stream or absence of typical shades), perspiring, and faintness.

The finding is made by trans-vaginal ultrasound assessment and can be affirmed by ectopic laparoscopy. Assuming that the finding is made early, clinical treatment utilizing the medication methotrexate might be thought of.

As a rule, a medical procedure which is generally a negligibly intrusive kind of medical procedure is expected to eliminate the pregnancy to save the existence of the lady.

On the off chance that blood loss is serious, blood transfusions are required. On the off chance that the ectopic pregnancy is situated in the Fallopian tube and because of that, if the Fallopian tube is impacted as the size of the undeveloped organism gets greater than the Fallopian tube must be eliminated on the off chance that it can't be fixed.

# Molar Pregnancy

This is a kind of pregnancy where cancer (development) creates from the placental tissue which doesn't permit the undeveloped organism (hatchling or kid) to typically be created.

A molar pregnancy might be noncancerous (hydatidiform mole) or may attack the mass of the belly (an intrusive mole).

A molar pregnancy that becomes dangerous is called choriocarcinoma.

On the off chance that the dead undeveloped organism and placental are not removed from the belly because of the intrusion of the mole, the dead tissue is known as a carneous mole.

The side effects and findings of molar pregnancy are equivalent to that of ectopic pregnancy.

The growth or mole can be eliminated by pull - (the expulsion of undesirable liquid material from the body with a needle and empty needle or with a gastrointestinal cylinder and a mechanical siphon), by D and C, or less usually by hysterectomy - (evacuation of the belly).

## Treatment Of Ectopic Pregnancy

The treatment choices are ordinarily evaluated after a pregnancy test and a trial of the chemical levels are found. Ultrasounds acted in the early weeks can assist with distinguishing the presence of one too.

Treatment choices will shift yet they all incorporate some type of end of the pregnancy.

Methotrexate is an infusion that can be offered assuming the pregnancy is in its earliest stage. This infusion forbids any further development and permits the pregnancy to end itself. This is the most non-intrusive of the choices. Careful expulsion or extension evacuation of the tissue is many times the strategy assuming the pregnancy has started to progress past the typical capacities of the methotrexate infusion.

Careful expulsion is done rapidly To save the mother further pain and take into account life-saving methods.

# Pregnancy After An Ectopic Pregnancy

Is it conceivable to get pregnant after you have experienced an ectopic pregnancy?

It is critical to have a causative variable distinguished to check whether there is another treatment you should take a stab at getting pregnant once more.

You might have to have a basic condition treated before thinking about another pregnancy. There is a background marked by certain ladies attempting to get pregnant after an ectopic pregnancy and conveying to term. Once more, be that as it may, different ladies can get pregnant.

# Why Can't The Ectopic Pregnancy Be Saved

The development of the egg will occur for a brief time frame. Nonetheless, any treated egg that has embedded itself along some unacceptable organ won't get the important supplements or the essential space it necessities to keep on developing. While comparing the prepared egg to cancer, the outcome is sincerely troublesome and can be comparative. As it develops it requests more space and at last will burst open the organ or organs that are confining its development. In addition to the fact that the mother ends up with super durable harm to the area, it can likewise confine or wipe out any possibilities of another pregnancy and it could too cost her life. Hence, an ectopic pregnancy can't be saved. Hence, it should be ended as soon as could be expected.

# How To Achieve Good Nutrition During Pregnancy

What would it be advisable for me to eat during pregnancy?  Stressed by accounts of how adding weight influences labor, numerous pregnant ladies need to understand what their sustenance (food) ought to contain.

This trepidation, many accept, is normal. For sure, a few inquiries frequently emerge when ladies are pregnant and are anticipating children. A portion of these inquiries are responded to here:

First and foremost, does a pregnant lady have to eat two times so a lot? It has frequently been said that a pregnant lady ought to eat for two individuals, yet this isn't correct. What is valid is that during pregnancy a lady needs to give great nourishment to two people. The developing child helps generally its sustenance from its mom through the umbilical rope, so diet is vital. Assuming the mother is deficient in any nutrients and supplements, her child could need them as well. In the event that a lady experienced difficulty keeping her weight up or down before the pregnancy, she ought to make a healthful arrangement with the assistance of her PCP or birthing specialist.

## How Much Energy Does A Woman Need During Pregnancy?

A lady who isn't pregnant necessities roughly 2,100 calories each day. A pregnant lady needs roughly 2,500 calories each day. A breastfeeding lady needs roughly 3,000 calories each day. Calories are once in a while called kilo-calories or kCals.

## What Sort Of Food Should Pregnant Woman Eat?

A decent equilibrium diet ought to contain something from all the food groups:

Dairy items,

Natural products,

Fish,

Vegetables,

Eggs,

Meat,

Fat and carbs.

A pregnant lady needs to eat something from every one of these nutritional categories consistently, to get legitimate measures of energy. Around 10% of calories ought to come from protein. Protein is essentially tracked down in meat, fish, eggs, dairy items, and beans. One more 35 percent of calories ought to come from fat, which is essentially tracked down in spread, oils, margarine, dairy items, and nuts, while 55% of calories ought to come from sugars, which are tracked down in bread, pasta, potatoes, rice, corn, and other grain items.

# What Other Vitamins And Minerals Are Essential During Pregnancy

They are folic acid, iron, zinc, and calcium.

## Folic Acid

During the initial three months of pregnancy (and ideally prior to becoming pregnant) a lady needs folic acid. This is one of the B-bunch nutrients and is otherwise called nutrient B9. It is significant during pregnancy for the creation of the child's sensory system. Folic acid can assist with forestalling brain tube imperfections, for example, spina bifida and other inborn deformities like a congenital fissure or congenital fissure.

Great normal wellsprings of folic acid are grain beans, natural products, green vegetables, squeezed orange, lentils, peas, and rice. It is suggested that all pregnant ladies take an everyday 400 micro gram supplement of folic corrosive daily for quite a long time, before origination and 90 days into their pregnancy.

The measurements of the enhancement ought to be bigger - 5mg each day - in the event that a lady has recently brought forth a youngster with a brain tube imperfection. On the off chance that she or her accomplice has spina bifida or family background of brain tube surrenders; or on the other hand assuming she has celiac illness (or other malabsorption states) diabetes mellitus, sickle cell pallor; or is taking anti-epileptic prescriptions. She ought to examine this matter with her PCP.

## Iron

During pregnancy, a lady's body needs more iron than expected to create all the blood expected to supply nourishment to the placenta. Great wellsprings of iron are green vegetables like broccoli and spinach, strawberries, mueshi, and wholemeal bread. Iron is all the more handily retained in the event that it is taken related to Vitamin C - either as an enhancement or in citrus natural products or juice. Tea and espresso can obstruct the body's retention of iron. It is in many cases suggested that all pregnant ladies take an iron enhancement consistently from the twentieth seven-day stretch of pregnancy.

This isn't required assuming a lady has a decent eating regimen and routine blood tests show that she isn't weak. Iron enhancements might cause blockage.

## Zinc And Calcium

These minerals, zinc, and calcium, are additionally required for the improvement of the incipient organism. Be that as it may, getting sufficient zinc and calcium by following a different diet is typically conceivable. Zinc and calcium can be gotten from eating fish like periwinkle and so on. Calcium is great for the child and mother's areas of strength.

# What Foods Should Be Avoided During Pregnancy

It is critical to stay away from Vitamin A during pregnancy since it might make harm the incipient organism. Food sources containing a lot of Vitamin An incorporate liver and ought to be eaten on an intermittent premise as it were. Unpasteurized cheddar, blue-veined cheeses, and pate are additionally not suggested as a result of the conceivable gamble of transmission of irresistible infections like listeria.

# How To Avoid Constipation During Pregnancy

Constipation during pregnancy can be made by hormonal changes that cause the digestive tract to move less. Iron enhancements can likewise cause obstruction. To stay away from clogging, eat loads of fiber-rich food sources like organic products, vegetables, wholemeal bread and cereal, prunes, and prune juice.

Drinking 2 to 3 liters of water every day will likewise assist with forestalling blockage by keeping stools damp. Customary activity will likewise assist with getting the digestion tracts going. Around 20 to 30 minutes of swimming or lively strolling a few times each week is a decent degree of activity to go for the gold. A drug specialist will want to give exhortation about OTC medications i.e Over-The-Counter arrangements that are protected to use during pregnancy to ease blockage.

# How Much Weight Should A Woman Gain During Pregnancy

It is viewed as ordinary to acquire 10 to 12kg (22 to 26lb). For down-to-earth reasons, the pregnancy is separated into three periods:

1. The main time frame runs from week 0 to 12 weeks where it is typical to acquire 1 to 2kg (2 to 4lb).

2. The subsequent period runs from week 12 to 28 weeks in which it is typical to acquire 300 to 400g (10 to 14oz) in seven days.

3. The third time frame runs from week 28 to 40 weeks and it is typical to acquire 1 to 3kg (2 to 6lb) a month.

Being over the top about your weight during pregnancy isn't required. Numerous obstetricians have quit gauging ladies other than at their most memorable visit on the grounds that the data is of little use in recognizing issues with the mother or her child.

Notwithstanding, overabundance weight gain is likely best stayed away from since most ladies will need to get back to a similar dress size inside a couple of long stretches of conveyance.

Where do the additional kilos come from?

An all-out weight increment of around 11.2kg (24lb) is typical.

A child weighs roughly 3.5kg (7lb 11oz) before birth.

The uterus develops to roughly 900g (11b 14oz).

The amniotic liquid weighs roughly 800g (1Lb 12oz).

The lady's bosoms develop by roughly 400g (14oz).

The heaviness of the additional blood is roughly 1.25kg (2Lb 12oz).

Water held in the body tissues weighs roughly 2kg (4 LB 60z).

The layer of fat underneath the skin weighs roughly 1.7kg (3Lb 11oz).

Each pregnant lady realizes that she can't consume fewer calories during her pregnancy. Be that as it may, what is the correct number of calories during pregnancy? Also, what are the best food sources to eat during pregnancy? What's more, are there food sources like feta cheddar and fish high in mercury that she should keep away from?

## Calories During Pregnancy

Pregnancy isn't an ideal opportunity to eat less, however, it is additionally not an opportunity to "eat for two". Weight gain during pregnancy should be without rushing and most ladies just need an extra 300 calories during pregnancy daily.

Obviously, in the event that you are finished or underweight, your consideration supplier, however, by and large, might have an alternate suggestion and hope to require an extra 300 calories per day. These additional calories will assist you with acquiring around 25 to 35 pounds during your pregnancy. That sounds like a great deal of weight, yet when you think about that the child will weigh 7 to 8 pounds, you can perceive that eating the legitimate measure of food and not a diet is so significant.

Increment of your bread and grains consumption.

Pregnant ladies ought to plan to have around 6 to 8 ounces (one ounce rises to one slice of bread) of grain sources a day. Grains give fiber and are high in iron and B nutrients. Preferably, pregnant ladies ought to intend to eat entire grains over different sorts of grains. Instead of nibbling on frozen yogurt, attempt a high fiber grain in milk with a sprinkle of cinnamon for a solid other option.

## Dairy and Calcium

A pregnant lady should get around 3 cups of dairy daily. Besides the fact that dairy contains calcium, which pregnant ladies do require, it likewise contains protein and Vitamins A, B-12, and D.

Great wellsprings of dairy items incorporate endlessly milk substitutes, sanitized cheddar, and yogurt.

In the event that you can't drink milk or could do without it, attempt soya milk or address your supplier about an extra wellspring of calcium. They might propose calcium-strengthened squeezed oranges, for instance.

Increase products of the soil consumption: Pregnant ladies should build their foods grown from the ground to four and a half cups a day. Leafy foods are high in fiber, nutrients A, C, and folic corrosive.

In a perfect world, you ought to get around 2 cups of leafy foods high in vitamin A and 2 cups high in Vitamin C, the other half cup ought to be your number one product of the soil. Leafy foods high in Vitamin An incorporate tomatoes, peaches, oranges, kiwi, peas, potatoes, spinach, squash and carrots.

# Protein Sources Safe To Eat During Pregnancy

Pregnant ladies need starches as well as protein. Meat and meat substitutes give pregnant ladies protein (counting most wellsprings of fish) that is protected to eat during pregnancy.

On the off chance that you are a veggie lover or a vegetarian, address your consideration supplier for an eating regimen custom-made to your necessities. Now that you are eating for at least two, this isn't an ideal opportunity to cut calories or hold off on junk food.

It is the polar opposite: you want around an additional 300 calories every day, particularly later in your pregnancy when your child develops rapidly. Assuming that you are extremely slim, exceptionally dynamic, or conveying products, you will require considerably more.

However, assuming you are overweight, your medical services supplier might exhort that you consume fewer additional calories.

Smart dieting is dependably significant, particularly when you are pregnant. So ensure your calories come from nutritious food varieties that will add to your child's development and improvement. Attempt to keep an even eating routine that consolidates the dietary rules:

Lean meats, natural products, vegetables, entire grain bread, and low-fat dairy items.

By eating a sound, adjusted diet you are bound to get the supplements you want. Be that as it may, you will require a greater amount of the fundamental supplements (particularly calcium, iron, and folic corrosive) than you did before you became pregnant.

Your medical services supplier will recommend pre-birth nutrients to be certain both you and your developing child are getting enough. Yet, taking pre-birth nutrients doesn't mean you can eat an eating regimen that is deficient in supplements. It is essential to recollect that you need to eat well while pregnant. Pre-birth nutrients are intended to enhance your eating routine not to be your main wellspring of much-required supplements.

## Calcium

Most ladies 19 years or more including individuals who are pregnant don't frequently get the day-to-day 1000mg of calcium that is suggested. Your developing child's calcium request is high subsequently, you are expected to expand your calcium utilization to keep a deficiency of calcium from your bones.

Your PCP will likewise logically endorse pre-birth nutrients for you which might contain some additional calcium. Great wellsprings of calcium incorporate low-fat dairy items including milk, sanitized cheddar, and yogurt, calcium-sustained items, including squeezed orange, soya milk, oats, dull green vegetables including spinach, kale, broccoli, tofu, dried beans, and almonds.

# Iron

Pregnant ladies need around 30 mg of iron each day, why? Since iron is expected to make hemoglobin, the oxygen-conveying part of the red platelets. The red platelets course all through the body to appropriate oxygen to all its cells.

Without enough iron, the body can't make sufficient red platelets, and the body's tissues and organs will not get the oxygen they need to work well. So every pregnant lady needs to get sufficient iron in her day-to-day diet, for her and the developing child in the belly.

Albeit the supplements can be found in different sorts of food varieties from meat sources are more effortlessly consumed by the body than the iron tracked down in plant food varieties.

Iron-improved food varieties incorporate Red meat, dim poultry salmon, eggs, tofu, enhanced grains, dried beans and peas, dried organic products, dim verdant green vegetables, blackstrap molasses, and iron-sustained breakfast oats.

# Health Tips On Drugs Intake

At the point when you are taking or drinking any medication don't consolidate it with blood medication since all blood-building drugs whether syrup (fluid), case, or tablet, contain a mineral known as iron that is fit for diminishing the force of the medication.  It is prudent, to take blood medication after the consummation of our medication measurement, e.g even jungle fever or antimicrobial medications. However, on the off chance that you are not happy or you are apprehensive, you can take your blood medication two after 2 hours as you drink your medications.

At the point when you drink your medications, stay away from the following;
1. Milk
2. Orange
3. Licking of Vitamin C
4. Drinking of Antacid (e.g, mismag)
5. Try not to blend blood tablets in with different medications (it will lessen the force of different medications as a result of their iron substance).
6. Stay away from kola nut.
7. Try not to eat coconut or hydrate.
8. Try not to consume your medications with tea, cold water, or sodas.

# Vaginal Hygiene

Vaginal diseases likewise can be brought about by nearby compounds or hypersensitive aggravations like the strategy for washing inside the vagina with cleanser, sudsy water or with some other fixing, or with filthy water. The vaginal can clean itself in light of the lactic corrosive and the peroxide it secretes, consequently don't utilize a cleanser. The cleanser likewise causes the broadening of the vaginal muscles. What's more, it can likewise make a few bubbles create in the vaginal. Kindly utilize clean water just for flushing. Try not to wear nylon pants.

Stay away from scented underwear liners and don't spray perfume on your vaginal. They all can cause diseases of positive and negative grams of miniature organic entities.

# Health Diagnosis

Many individuals both old and youthful, including kids are kicking the bucket regularly because the patients (individuals) need to be prudent or perhaps they need to deal with their cash. Yet, in no time, the circumstance turns out to be most terrible.

Each time you are not feeling great, you are supposed to go to the emergency clinic for a conclusion or to a certified clinical research center to run your blood test to discover the foundations for potential treatment. Yet many individuals like to purchase medications to drink without having the information on the reasons for their disorders or illnesses, they are drinking the medications. Kindly, see your PCP before it is past the point of no return in an instance of any disorder or contamination assault. Try not to drink indiscriminately.

# Ulcer Patients

Ulcer Patients ought to keep away from pineapple and orange or they ought to take nearly nothing. These organic products will in general deteriorate the ulcer and the agonies. Ulcer patients shouldn't drink acid neutralizers along with the ulcer tablets for example (Cimetidine, or Omeprazole ), till the following 2 hours, after ingesting the medications. On the off chance that not the stomach settling agent (for example Mismag, Gestid, Gascol, Supermag e. t. c) is fit for decreasing the power or adequacy of the medication. Assuming you have a duodenum ulcer or gastric ulcer, It is a cimetidine drug that is great for you. Yet, assuming it is a peptic ulcer, it is an omeprazole drug that is great for you. Ensure you deworm yourself and your kids like clockwork. Combantrin (Pyrantel Pamoate) is great for you. It crushes the worms.

# Kidney Stones Problems and Solutions

The kidney is the organ that channels the blood and discharges (byproducts) an abundance of water from the body as pee. The kidneys are situated at the rear of the stomach depression, of the gut, on one or the other side of the spine. There is a typical insight about the torment of kidney stones. Anybody who has at any point encountered the agony of kidney stones would understand what I am referring to. It is an agonizing aggravation. It is an aggravation like no other. This sort of aggravation is many times on one side of the mid-region, emanating down into the stomach or the genital region. Now and again there is queasiness and heaving.

## What Is A Kidney Stone

A kidney stone is a hard, translucent mineral material framed inside the kidney or urinary plot. Kidney stones will generally create from squander matter solidifying and becoming joined to within the mass of the kidney and may stay inconspicuous until the issue is extreme. Kidney stones are shaped when there is a lessening in pee volume and an overabundance of stone-framing substances in the pee.

# Why The Pain

The kidney is creating pee however it can't get pushed down. The stone blocks the progression of pee, causing a reinforcement. The framework is attempting to push pee out from the kidneys and the stone is obstructing it, causing serious agonies. This is called hydronephrosis, it goes back and forth and it is very agonizing because you are extending your framework.

Adjacent to the flank torment there could be blood in the pee moreover.

Most kidney stones stay inconspicuous until removed, getting found out in a ureter or other entryway while traveling through the body during pee.

# Causes Of Kidney Stones

There are sure infections and conditions related to kidney stones, including corpulence and diabetes. In the event that you don't hydrate or you are enamored with enjoying high salt admission and an eating routine wealthy in creature protein, it makes your pee ferment, and afterward, you could turn out to be more inclined to have kidney stones.

Likewise in the event that you have a family background of kidney stones, you are more able to get a kidney stone.

After you have had a kidney stone, you are bound to have one again except if you go to preventive lengths as made sense of above or prior.

# Diagnosis And Treatment

Determination isn't convoluted however specialists generally suggest a CT check as the best quality level for diagnosing kidney stones. It isn't possible convincingly from a blood test anything more. Assuming that the kidney stones are adequately little, they typically drop all alone. At times it very well may be an unremarkable section, or once in a while it is only a difficult entry, however, analgesics (torment ease medications) and a few different prescriptions can help.

Frequently kidney stones bigger than 5mm may require careful activity or expulsion. In any case, you unquestionably don't need that since it is obtrusive, tedious, and costly. So the most ideal way is to contract the kidney stone, break it, or stay away from it through and through.

# Treatment And Prevention

There are basic, reasonable approaches to staying away from the aggravation of kidney stones utilizing normal spices and food varieties either to lighten an extensive variety of kidney problems or to reestablish renal action. It starts with drinking enough water routinely and avoiding diets (food) wealthy in creature fat.

# Apple Cider Vinegar

Drinking apple juice vinegar assists with changing the body's pH worth and it additionally assists with laying out a basic shaping state in the pee. Uric corrosive, the synthetic liable for the arrangement of gout gems and urate kidney stones can't take shape in

## New Lemon Fruit

Lemonades are high in citrate. The juice of new lemons is sufficiently able to break up particular sorts of kidney stones, and drinking lemon water can assist with exploiting these advantages. Crush new lemon organic product with water and drink up to 2 liters of this blend spread over the day for ordinarily inside couples of certain weeks.

## Marshmallow Root

Is known for getting urethritis and aiding flushing kidney stones. It produces adhesive, a thin. mucus film that covers the urinary lot as well as the whole intestinal system, safeguarding the coating from progressing attacks from poisons. You can accept it as natural tea. You can see them in drug stores and general store shops.

## Cranberry Juice

It is high in supplements, for example, anthocyanins, L-ascorbic acid, and cancer prevention agents. Some unsweetened cranberry concentrate blended in with 3 cups of water, can be over the day for each day for certain weeks. You can improve it with honey assuming you like.

## Parsley And Dandelion

New parsley and dandelion greens are spices popular for their uncommon restorative properties for easing urinary lot issues. Both are normal diuretics (assist with eliminating overabundance of water from the body), animating urinary results, and flushing the arrangement of waste materials that add to the development of kidney stones. They eliminate poisons, purify the kidney, disintegrate uric corrosive, and establish a basic framing climate in the kidneys and bladder, assisting the pee with keeping an impartial or marginally soluble pH. You can utilize parsley and dandelion as tea or hack and add them to your plates of mixed greens.

# Poor Blood Circulation Causes And Solutions

Circulatory issues don't start in a day. As such, you could call the heart an exceptionally tolerant organ, which can require long stretches of misuse and when it can't take it any longer it breaks out.

## Causes Of Poor Blood Circulation

Unfortunate blood flow is a result of a specific way of life decisions that certain individuals make that are thus negative or risky to their well-being.

Combined with these are factors like an imbalanced eating regimen and actual activity. This large number of variables and a lot more prompt greasy stores on the blood vessel walls, which then solidified into what is called plaque. These plaques then, at that point, hinder or make obstacles to the smooth section of blood to and from the heart.

Plaques consume a large chunk of the day to be shaped, that is the explanation, we find circulatory issues influencing the typical age individuals and the old more frequently than they influence kids.

Our food propensities likewise add to an unfortunate development of cholesterol which might build the consistency of the blood, which again makes trouble or inconsistency in the smooth move through corridors and veins.

# Symptoms Of Poor Blood Circulation

Since the circulatory framework covers the whole body, the issues can likewise appear in various ways.

## Mind

The mind gets 20% of the blood course in the body. With a drop in the progression of blood, the mind's capabilities are poor, bringing about feeling torpid - - (sleepiness or sluggish), loss of memory, absence of mental cause, and so forth.

Successive unexplained migraines and abrupt assaults of dazedness are likewise viewed as side effects of unfortunate blood dissemination to the cerebrum.

## Heart

At the point when unfortunate blood flow influences the heart, the side effects would be chest torment, hypertension, and ascend in the degree of cholesterol. Trouble in playing out any normal errand like climbing steps, or strolling a stretch could make you exceptionally drained and winded.

## Liver

At the point when you experience the ill effects of an absence of hunger or experience abrupt weight reduction and your skin looks drab - (dull and lacking brilliance), it is very conceivable that your liver is getting 'languid' and these are the early side effects of unfortunate blood dissemination to the liver.

## Kidneys

This organ assumes a significant part in directing and observing the circulatory strain other than taking out the waste and overabundance of water from the body.

At the point when unfortunate blood flow influences the kidneys, you will see enlargement of hands, feet and lower legs, ascend in circulatory strain - (hypertension), adjusted pulse, and feel tired constantly. Unfortunate blood dissemination likewise, can cause hypertension.

## Appendages

Unfortunate blood flow can genuinely affect the arms and legs. You might encounter abrupt deadness of the hands, feet, and fingers or experience difficult leg cramps.

Side effects of serious blood course issues can be varicose veins or a condition called stenosis - (which is when a piece of the skin becomes blue or dark because of an absence of sufficient oxygen to the concerned tissues).

## Sex Drive

Unfortunate blood course can influence the conceptive organs. The side effects are the absence of sex drive and fatigue (sleepiness).

Side effects would likewise incorporate the absence of imperativeness (strength). Serious blood dissemination issues could make somebody barren moreover.

# Prevention Of Poor Blood Circulation

1. Eat an adjusted diet

2. Foster a solid way of life

3. Do actual activity occasionally

4. Keep away from low-thickness lipoproteins (LDL) cholesterol. Eg, spread and so on.

5. Foster a good food propensity

6. Additionally, take food supplements like vitamin B-complex, astyfer, astymin, and so forth.

# Treatment

Each grown-up from the age of 20 years should begin going for a cholesterol clinical examination at spans among different tests.

Whenever found that the cholesterol is high, drugs like statins will be endorsed by the clinical specialist. These medications can't be taken in any case since they make side impacts.

# Anemia

This is a condition where the centralization of the oxygen conveying shade hemoglobin in the blood is beneath typical.  Hemoglobin particles are conveyed inside red platelets and they transport oxygen from the lungs to the tissues.  Typically, stable hemoglobin focuses in the blood are kept up with by harmony between red cell creation in the bone marrow and red cell obliteration in the spleen. Sickliness might result, assuming this equilibrium is vexed or unusual. Frailty isn't an illness but a component of many problems.

## Types OF Anemia

There are different kinds of frailty, which can be grouped into those because of diminished or faulty red cell creation by the bone marrow. In this subject, the focus is based on the faulty red platelet creation by the bone marrow. In this condition, the body comes up short on the measure of red platelets to stay aware of the body's interest in oxygen. Figuring out the various orders of weakness can assist us with perceiving the side effects and keep away from pallor issues.

## Iron Deficiency Anemia

Lack of iron paleness is a condition wherein the body has too minimal iron in the circulation system.  This type of iron deficiency is more normal in grown-ups and ladies before menopause. Blood misfortune from weighty feminine periods, inward draining from the gastrointestinal lot, or giving a lot of blood can all add to this condition.

Different causes can be unfortunate dietary propensities or persistent digestive illnesses. The signs and side effects are whiteness, cerebral pain, and peevishness. Side effects of more extreme lack of iron pallor include: - Dyspnea (suspension of breath or powerlessness to breathe well), fast heartbeat (palpitation), and weak hair and nails.

## Treatment

Treatment typically appears as oral iron enhancements and dietary changes.

## Folic Deficiency Anemia

This sort of weakness is otherwise called megaloblastic sickliness. This type of paleness is described by an absence of folic corrosive, one of the B-complex gathering of nutrients, in the circulatory system.

This is typically brought about by a deficient admission of folic corrosive, normally tracked down in vegetables. However, on the off chance that the vegetables are overcooked, you will free or obliterate the folic corrosive substance.

Liquor addiction can likewise be a contributing variable here of frailty. During pregnancy when the folic corrosive is utilized more or in the early stages, this condition can likewise show itself.

It can likewise be caused as a symptom of other blood problems.

The side effects of this condition or confusion are shortcomings, fatigue (sleepiness), memory slips (misfortune), and touchiness.

## Treatment

This condition can be tried not by incorporating food sources with folic corrosive in the eating regimen or you can get it to drink as a tablet. Such food sources include hamburgers, liver, asparagus, and red beans.

# Noxious Anemia

Noxious weakness generally influences individuals between the ages of 50 and 60 years or more because of the absence of vitamin B12.

This illness can be genetic, yet a few types of the condition can be autoimmune infections. Individuals who have autoimmune infections are bound to have a malicious weakness.

Side effects of this type of paleness include fatigue, dyspnea, heart palpitations, deadness, or shivering at the furthest points.

# Aplastic Anemia

Aplastic iron deficiency is brought about by nonattendance or a decrease in red platelets. This can occur through injury where the blood-forming tissue in the bone marrow is obliterated. Along these lines, the victim can't battle disease and is probably going to be a weighty bleeder.

Side effects include Lethargy (a sensation of sluggishness tiredness, or absence of energy), pallor, and purpura (a gathering of problems described by purplish or rosy earthy colored regions or spots of discoloration brought about by dying) inside the skin or mucous films. Purpura likewise alludes to a stained region of the body) dying, quick heartbeat, diseases, and congestive cardiovascular breakdown.

There is no clear known reason for aplastic iron deficiency, yet it is believed to be brought about by openness to specific poisons and hepatitis infection.

## Sickle Cell Anemia

This type of paleness is of an inherited sort and is a consequence of an unusual kind of red platelets. Sickle cell paleness is a dangerous infection and there is no counteraction.

Side effects of this condition include: agonizing assault on arms, legs, and stomach, jaundice in the whites of the eyes, fever, extreme fatigue (shortcoming), quick heartbeat, pallor.

Intricacies include leg ulcers, shock, cerebral drain, and muscular (bones) messes.

## Polycythemia Vera

This illness is more normal in moderately aged men and is described by an expansion in red platelets, leucocytes, and thrombocytes. There is an extremely quick and serious multiplication of cells and the bone marrow cells mature more quickly than expected. The reason for this condition is obscure.

Side effects are Purplish shaded skin, ragged-looking eyes, cerebral pain, wooziness, and expanded spleen.

Albeit the signs and side effects of iron deficiency might appear to be overpowering, fortunately, most structures can be controlled with medicine furthermore, dietary changes.

# Stroke And The Causes

A stroke is a harm to the piece of the mind made to interfere with its blood supply. The interference is most frequently caused by the blockage of a cerebral corridor by blood coagulation, which might have been conveyed into the conduit in the dissemination from coagulation somewhere else in the body. Stroke may likewise result from restricted discharge because of a crack of a vein in or close to the mind. The rate of stroke increases with age and is higher in men.

Certain elements increment the gamble. The most significant are hypertension and atherosclerosis (and by affiliation, factors, for example, smoking that add to these problems). Other gamble factors are atrial fibrillation (a harmed heart valve), and a new cardiovascular failure (myocardial dead tissue), these can cause clumps in the heart which might relocate to the mind.

Because of the persevering deficient course of blood and oxygen to the mind because of the blockage of the veins by blood cluster or cholesterol (immersed fat, for example, margarine) the issue created from such a condition is called stroke (loss of motion). A stroke could be incomplete or an out stroke.

## Symptoms

Symptoms generally grow abruptly and, contingent upon the size, causes, and degree of cerebrum harm may include: migraine, dazedness, visual unsettling influence, development, or capability constrained by the harmed region of the mind is weakened. Shortcoming or loss of motion on one side of the body is called hemiplegia-(this is a typical impact of a serious stroke). A stroke that influences the predominant cerebral half of the globe might cause an unsettling influence on the language. This is a sort of stroke called aphasia. This sort of stroke prompts a total shortfall of recently gained language abilities, brought about by a cerebrum problem that influences the capacity to talk and compose or the capacity to talk and compose or the capacity to fathom or (comprehend) and read.

Language capability in the mind lies in the predominant cerebral half of the globe. Two specific regions on this side of the equator are Broca's and Wernicke's regions and the pathways associating the two, are significant in language abilities.

Harm to these areas, which most generally happens because of stroke or head injury can prompt aphasia. The more extreme the aphasia, the less the possibilities of recuperation.

About 33% of significant strokes are deadly, the third outcome in some handicap, and a third make no enduring sick impacts. Ischemia kind of stroke results from inadequate blood supply to a particular organ or tissue. This type is generally brought about by illness of the veins like atherosclerosis, however, may likewise result from injury, tightening (decrease in size) of a vein because of fit of the muscles in the vessel wall, or lacking blood stream because of wasteful siphoning of the heart.

Side effects rely upon the area impacted. Treatment might incorporate vasodilator medications to broaden the veins or in additional serious cases, angioplasty or sidestep activity might be completed.

## Diagnosis And Treatment

At times critical treatment might work on the possibilities of recuperation. ECG (electrocardiogram), CT check, chest X-beams, blood tests, angiography-(imaging that empowers veins to be seen on X-beam film), and MRI (attractive reverberation imaging) might be utilized to examine the reason and degree of cerebrum harm. On the off chance that a stroke is demonstrated by sweep to be because of apoplexy (blood clump), thrombolytic medications might be given.

Anticoagulants might be given on the off chance that there is a conspicuous wellspring of an embolism (blockage of the corridor by cluster), like atrial fibrillation or a restricted carotid conduit. Now and again, anti platelet specialists, for example, headache medicine are given. As a rule, regard for hydration and strain regions, and great nursing care, are the main effects on the result. Physiotherapy might reestablish lost development or sensation, language instruction might help language aggravations.

# Conclusion

In conclusion, we hope this guide has given you a solid foundation in the basics of health and wellness. Remember that good health is a journey, not a destination, and it takes time and effort to make positive changes.

By making small, sustainable changes to your nutrition, exercise, sleep, and mental health habits, you can improve your overall well-being and enjoy a happier, healthier life. And if you're struggling with a chronic condition or navigating the healthcare system, don't be afraid to seek support from healthcare professionals or loved ones.

Always remember that taking care of yourself is a top priority, and with the knowledge and tools provided in Health Basics 101, you can take the first step towards a healthier, happier you. Here's to your continued health and wellness!